AF261445

Flustered Without Mustard
Finding Calm When Angry or Frustrated

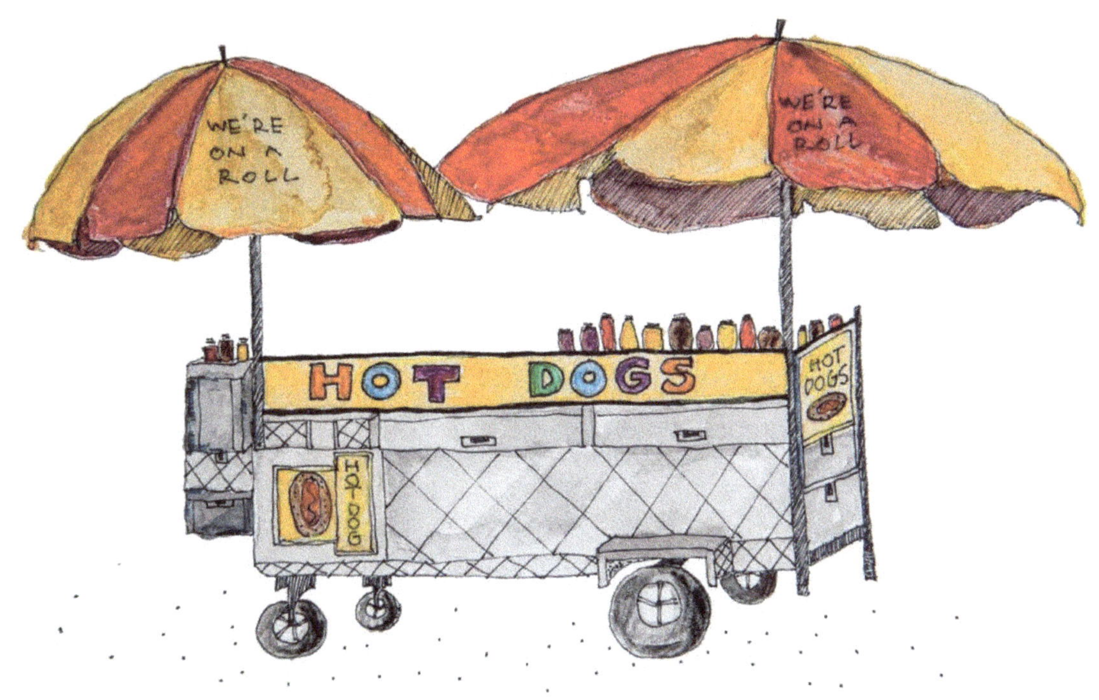

Word Wranglin' by Barbara 'Rhubarb' Haas
Wondrous Watercolors by Mary Ann 'June Hog' Kruse

Flustered Without Mustard
Finding Calm When Angry or Frustrated

Published by Rhubarb Wisdom Books
Text copyright © 2020 by Barbara ˝Rhubarb˝ Haas

Illustrations copyright © 2020 by Mary Ann ˝JuneHog˝ Kruse
Artwork by JuneHog Designs:
https://www.redbubble.com/people/junehog/shop

Creative Market Fonts: BookWorm & My Dear Watson
Photos of Illustrations: Dave Kozlowski Photography

Library of Congress Control Number: 2020910067

Paperback ISBN: 978-0-578-68073-6
Hardcover ISBN: 978-1-7350831-0-0

RhubarbWisdomBooks.com
For permission or to contact the author/publisher:
RhubarbWisdomBooks@gmail.com

"Granma said when you come on something good,
first thing to do is share it with whoever you can find:
that way the good spreads out to where no telling it will go."

The Education of Little Tree
by Forrest Carter

"As we shall see, listening to stories while looking at
pictures stimulates children's deep brain networks,
fostering their optimal cognitive development."

*The Enchanted Hour: The Miraculous
Power of Reading Aloud in the Age of Distraction*
by Meghan Cox Gurdon

Dedication

To our niece, Ivee Ann, who loves books

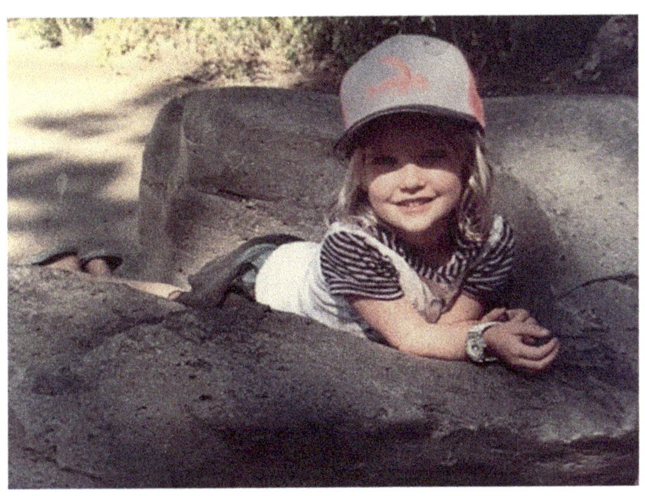

To our parents, Ivee's grandparents,
Killian Nicholas & Patricia Ann Kruse

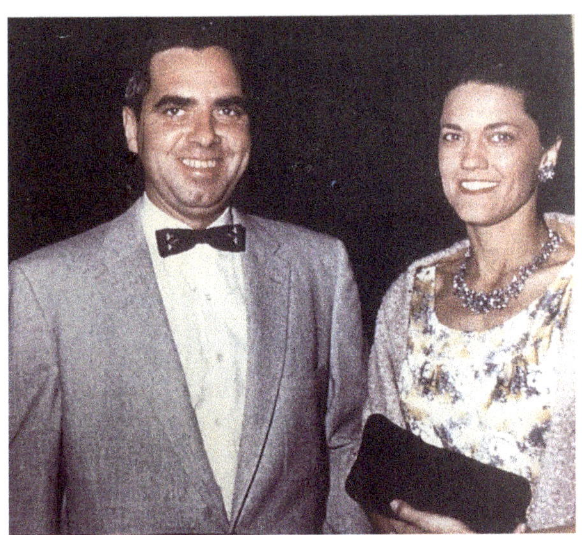

Preface

Welcome to Rhubarb Wisdom Books!

Why Rhubarb?

My dad called me Rhubarb throughout his life with a smile and a twinkle in his eye, and it made me feel special. During my teaching career this helped me to understand the importance of finding and developing a connection with each student. Thanks, Dad.

What is a Wisdom Book?

In my classroom I called any book with a lesson, a moral, or insight a wisdom book. As a youngster I yearned for lessons that were beyond reading, writing, and arithmetic. Nowadays students are taught character-building and emotional intelligence skills as part of the basic curriculum and receive the kinds of wisdoms I longed for in my school years.

A Master of Arts in Education and many courses over four decades taught me how to blend the science of teaching with the art of teaching. Brain-based learning methods incorporate images to engage the brain and create more meaning, so I used picture books to introduce various topics. The books sparked interest, motivated learning, and prompted thinking. Quotes from wisdom books were used to instigate lively and heartwarming discussions, improve writing, and encourage points to ponder about the students' own highly individualized curriculums in life.

Why are Big Breaths Important?

As a child when I was in the midst of any meltdown, my mom's advice was always to 'take three big breaths.' Research shows that taking deep, slow breaths helps to focus on present awareness, reduces anxiety, and relieves stress. Schools and households around the world are enjoying the benefits of this mindfulness technique. Thanks, Mom.

Why read *Flustered Without Mustard: Finding Calm When Angry or Frustrated?*

This rhyming picture book is about a hot dog vendor without mustard and a wide variety of his customers' reactions. The words and illustrations share ideas to consider when faced with unexpected situations, and concepts to help take responsibility for one's own emotions. The story has two sections to allow more flexibility for discussions.

Acknowledgments

"I am the only person who has the power to decide what I will be.
I make myself what I am." - Marva Collins, innovative inner city teacher

It was delightful to collaborate with my artsy sister extraordinaire, Mary Ann, on the illustrations. May her drawings bring a twinkle to your eyes, and help you remember ways to calm and tap into your own inner strengths and wisdom.

I am grateful for the encouragement and suggestions from my husband, Chris, my siblings and extended family, and many friends while writing this wisdom book of my own.

I am thrilled and honored to have testimonials for this book from artists, authors, educators, and counselors with such expertise in their fields.

Many thanks to all the students from elementary to graduate level that I have taught or mentored, and to the parents, fellow teachers, and professors I have worked with through the years. You have enriched my life in many ways, and what I have learned from you has been inspiring and meaningful.

The Marva Collins' quote above was part of my classroom's Daily Pledge. It brings me memories of smiling youngsters with strong voices full of hopes and dreams. Ms. Collins understood the importance of emotional development, and the long lasting consequences of any shame-based ways in education. She encouraged her students to focus on their unique talents and on improvement, that education wasn't only about straight As in all subjects. She realized that emotional and academic progress are connected and important for a more balanced life.

Thank you to Brene' Brown's *Daring Greatly*, Esther Hicks', *Getting Into the Vortex Relationship Guided Meditation*, Sandra Ingerman's *How to Heal Toxic Thoughts*, Harriet Lerner's *Dance of Anger* and *Dance of Connection*, Marshall Rosenberg's *Non-Violent Communication*, and Marianne Williamson's *Return to Love*. These books offered me the practical tools I needed to better understand my own emotions, and helped me to guide my students more effectively when dealing with their own wide range of feelings.

Flustered Without Mustard
Finding Calm When Angry or Frustrated

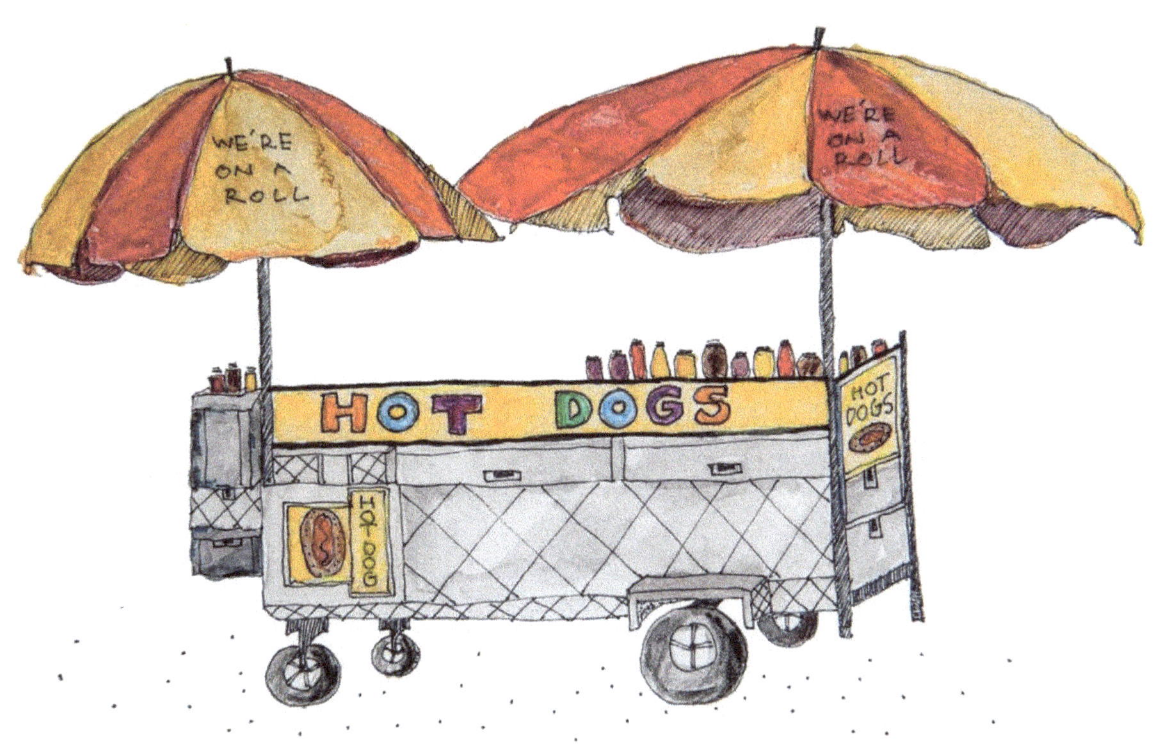

Word Wranglin' by Barbara 'Rhubarb' Haas

Wondrous Watercolors by Mary Ann 'June Hog' Kruse

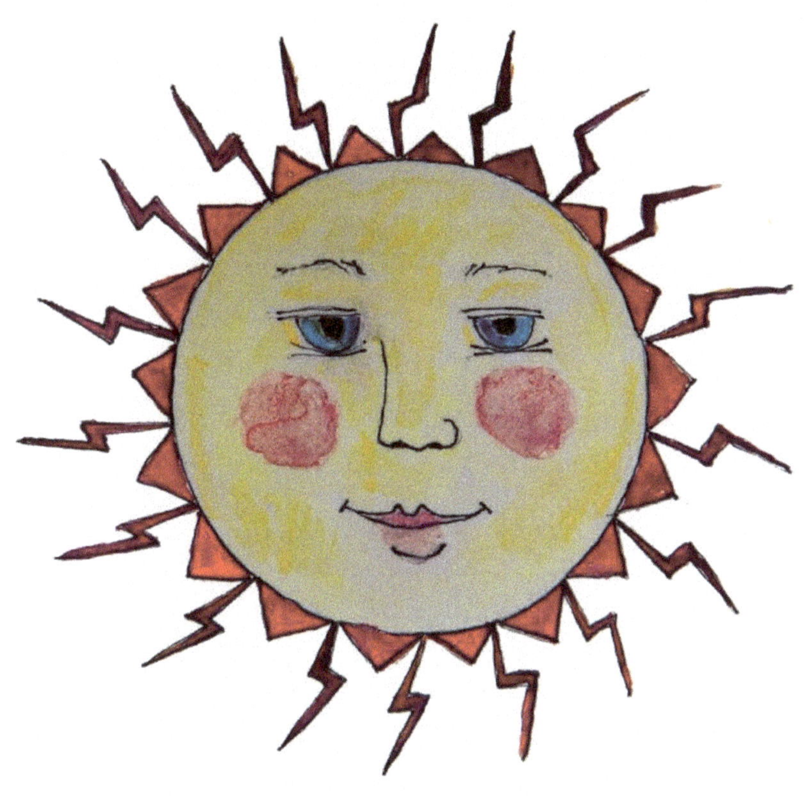

"It's a beautiful Sunday! I'm feeling 'sahweeeet'!

I'm cooking up hot dogs for everyone to eat!

My cart's all ready! I've got customers to greet!"

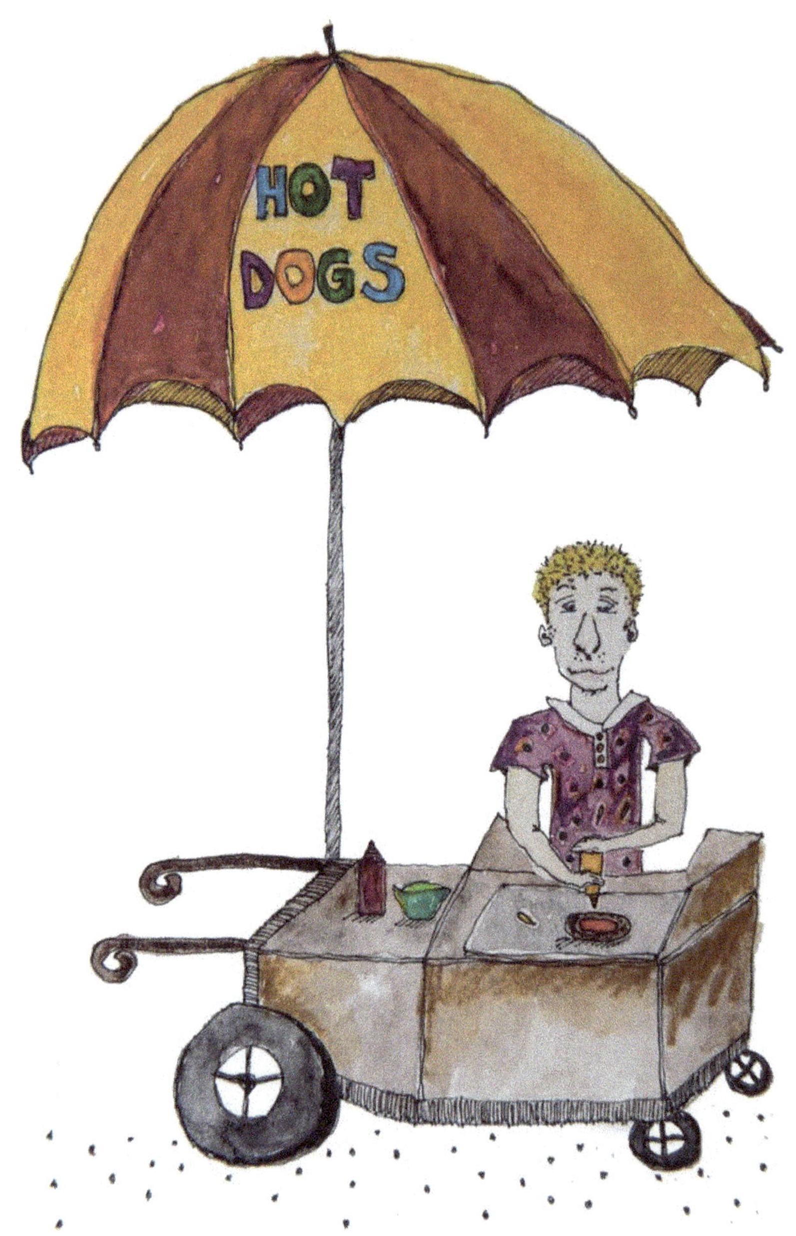
HOT
DOGS

Then later that afternoon . . .

The hot dog vendor, boom, ran out of mustard.
He felt really bad, and was really flustered.

This lack of mustard set things in motion.
There were lessons learned, many thoughts, notions.

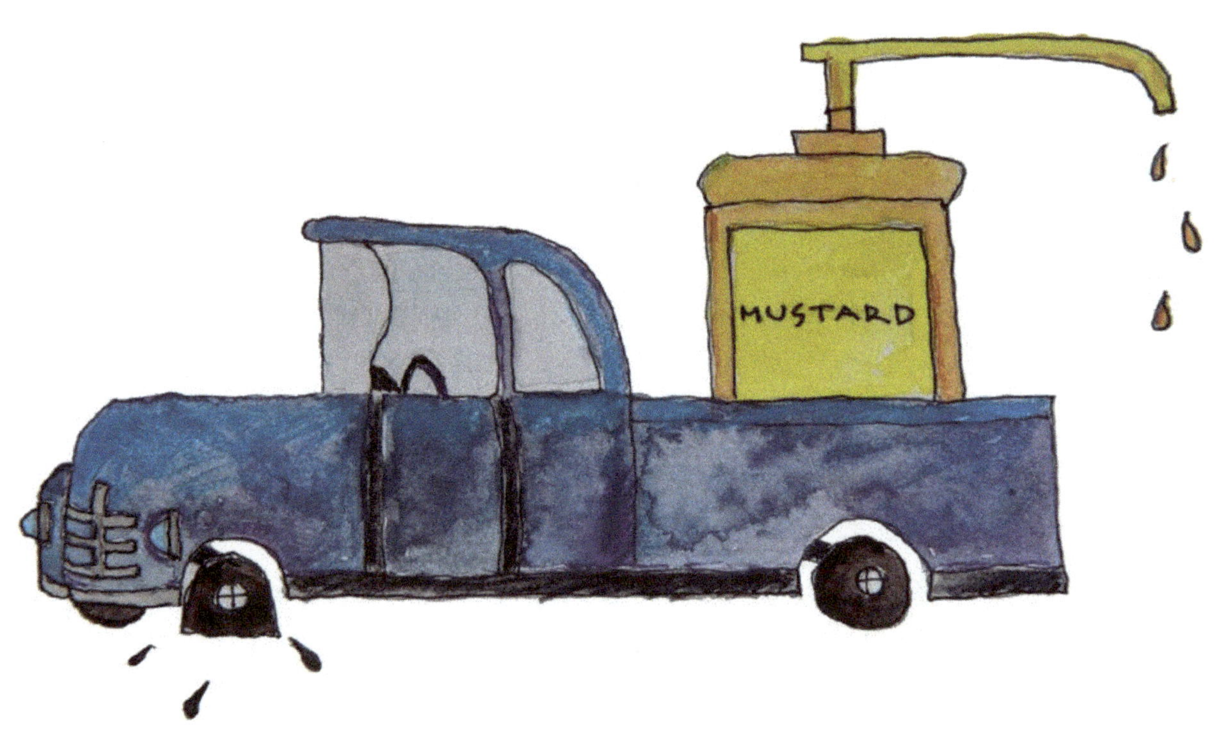
MUSTARD

The vendor ran out of mustard that day.
He had ordered early, no thoughts of delay.

Next time he'll order even more than before.
He appreciated his customers & now many felt sore.

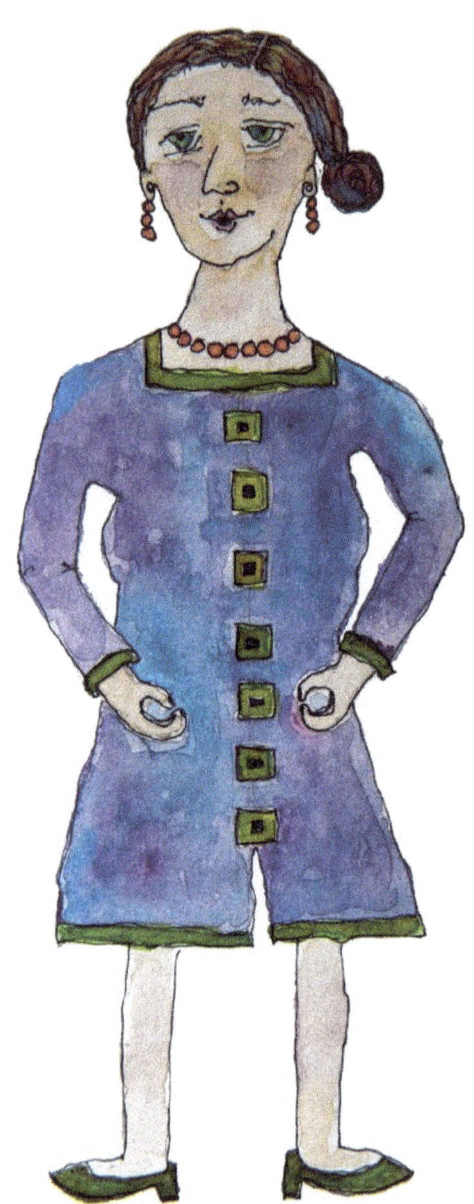

One woman was mad, felt really disappointed.
She started screaming, her finger pointed.

She suddenly realized she was starting to blame,
That anger towards others was not a fair game.

She apologized, her voice starting to crack.
"I'm so sorry, I need to breathe, and not attack."

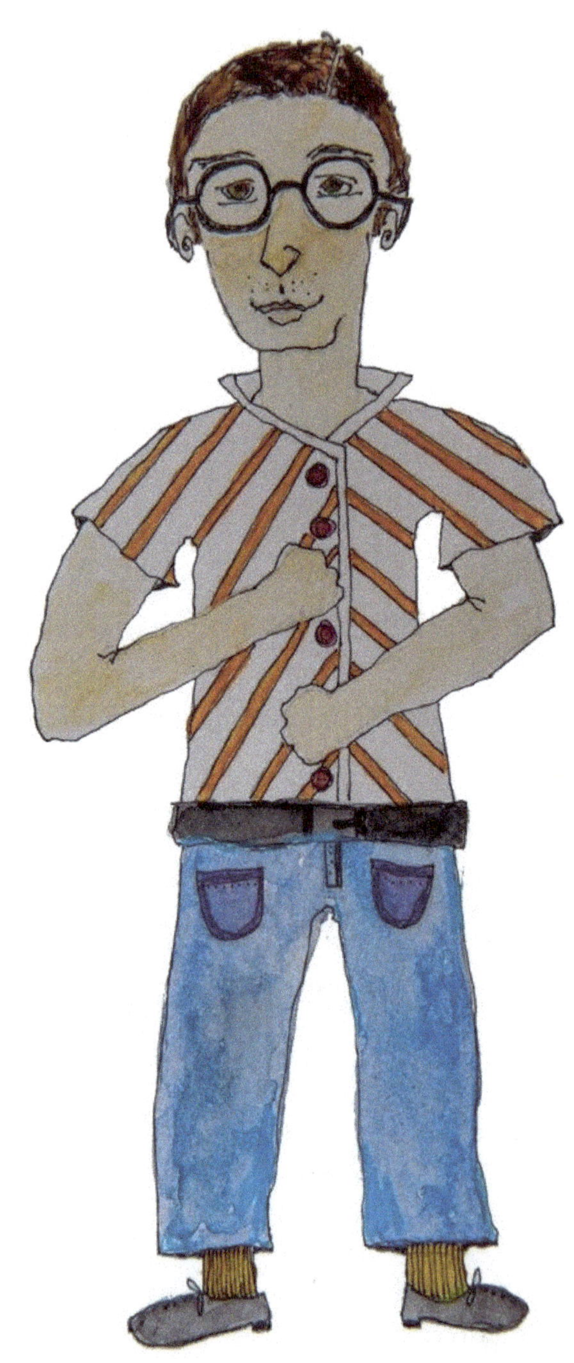

A man raised his fist to hit the cart of the vendor.
He wanted to act out instead of surrender.

He paused and remembered to drum on his belly.
Until he mellowed out, he just wiggled like jelly.

He found some control before he did strike.
"Whew, I'm proud I chose not to be warlike."

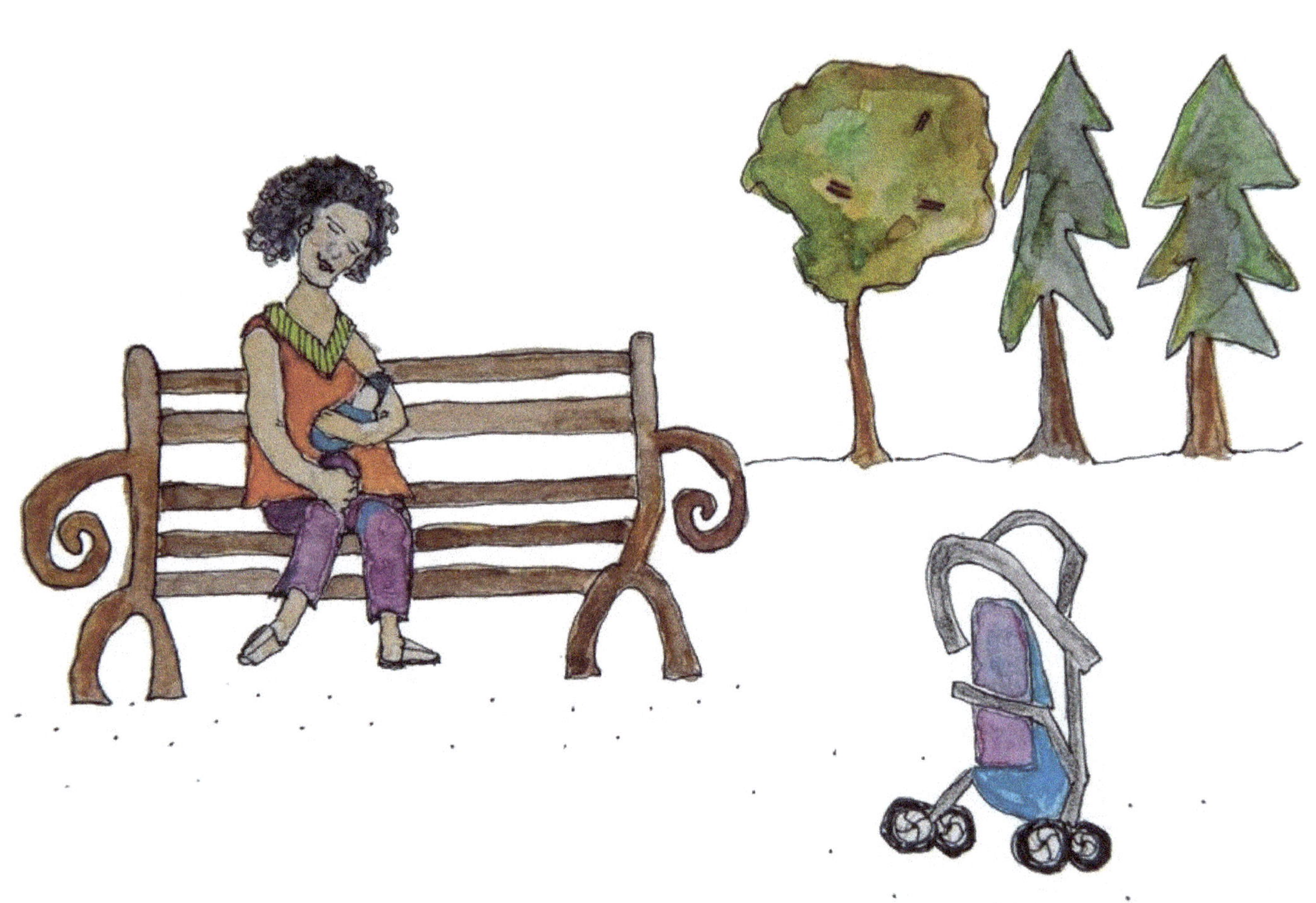

A mom heard the news, then broke down and wept.
She was overwhelmed already, so was easily upset.

She strolled to a park to sit in the sun,
Closed her eyes to relax holding her little loved one.

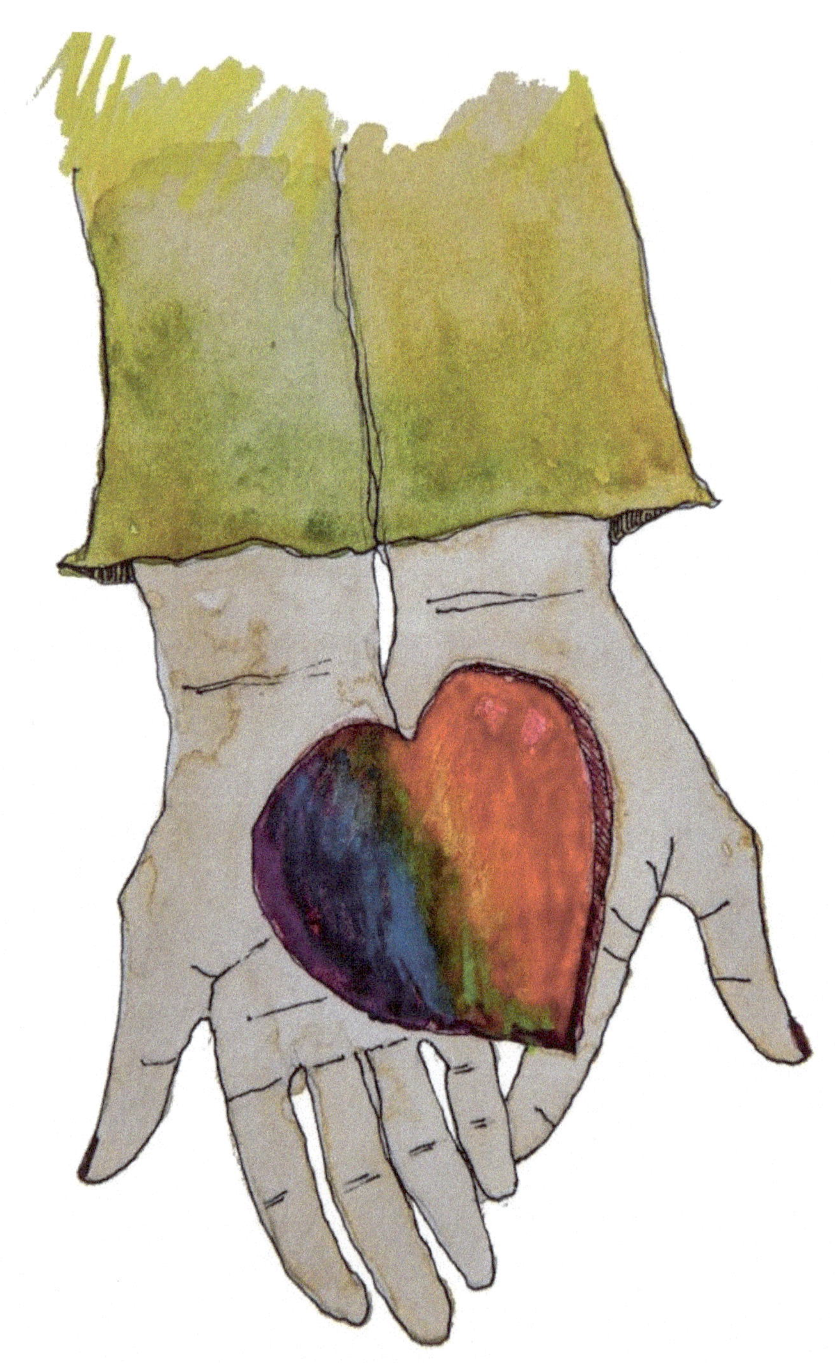

She thought of puppies, kittens, rainbows, & sunsets.
She took time to calm down, no reacting, no regrets.

With images of innocence and hands on her heart,
Quieting her mind was so needed, so smart.

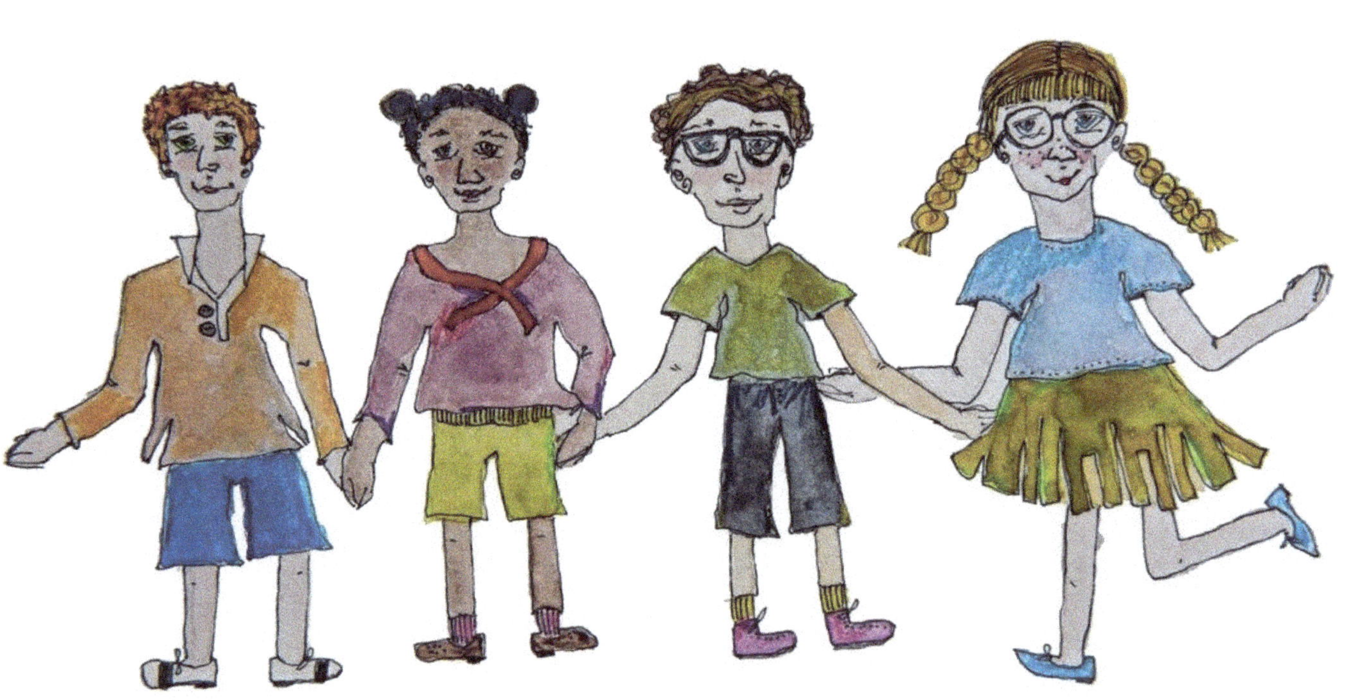

Some teens wanted mustard, so decided to leave.
They walked & talked more, 'stead of stay and grieve.

They knew there would be other vendors somewhere.
They used friendship for guidance & did not despair.

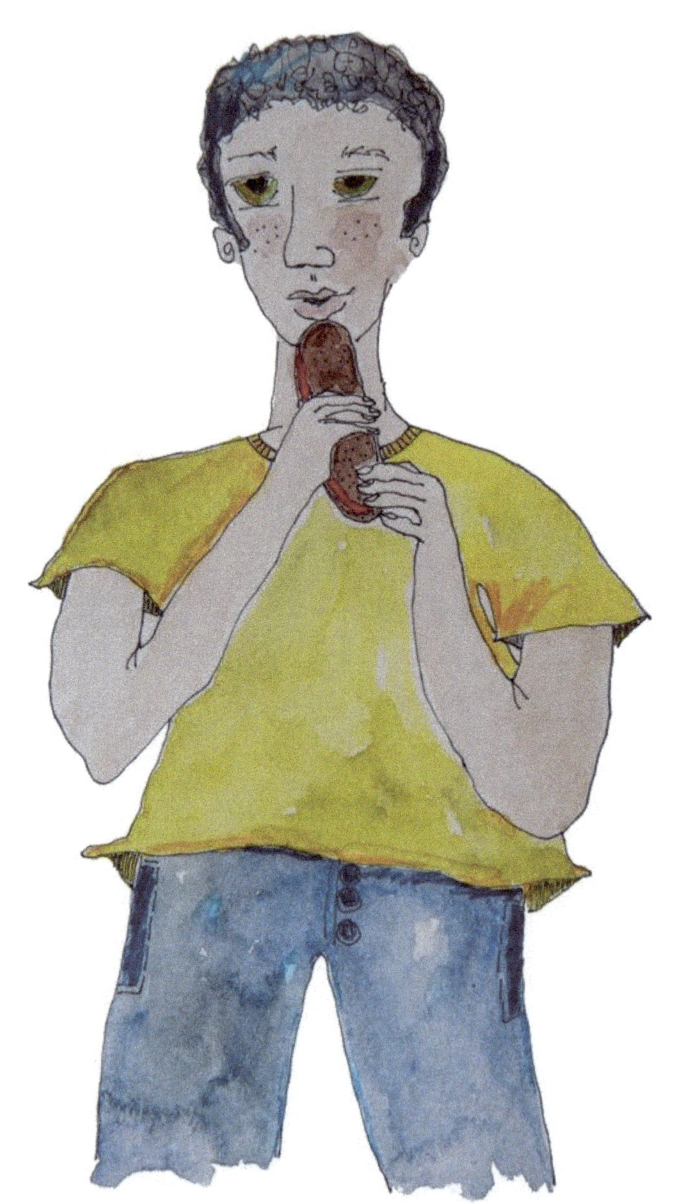

A boy usually ordered "with mustard, please."
Yet, was quite hungry, so munched it up with ease.

He stayed cool, calm, collected, & thought it wise
To send kindness to the vendor, looking into his eyes.

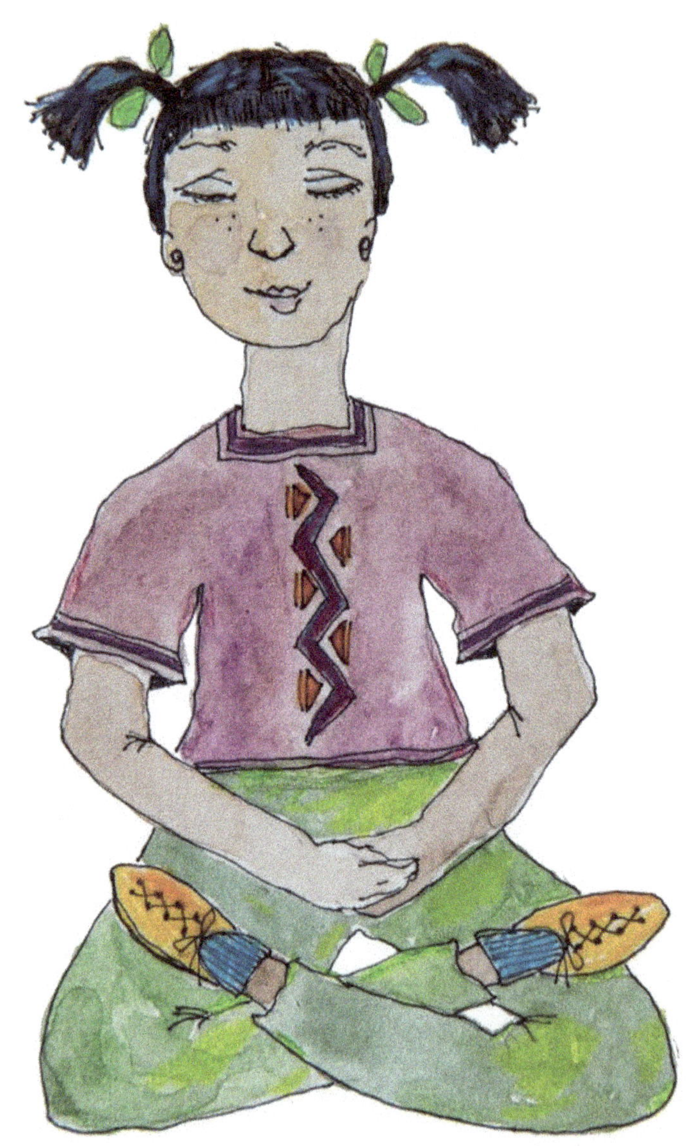

Folks faulted the vendor for his miscalculations.
They felt sad or mad with unmet expectations.

Some were offended, went off like a bomb.
Many missed that mustard, and found ways to calm.

Taking three big breaths in moments of strife,
Can help when you're angry or flustered in life.

To practice breathe slowly now 1 . . . 2 . . . 3 . . .
Ahhh! This sweet place of mellow will set you free!

* * * * *

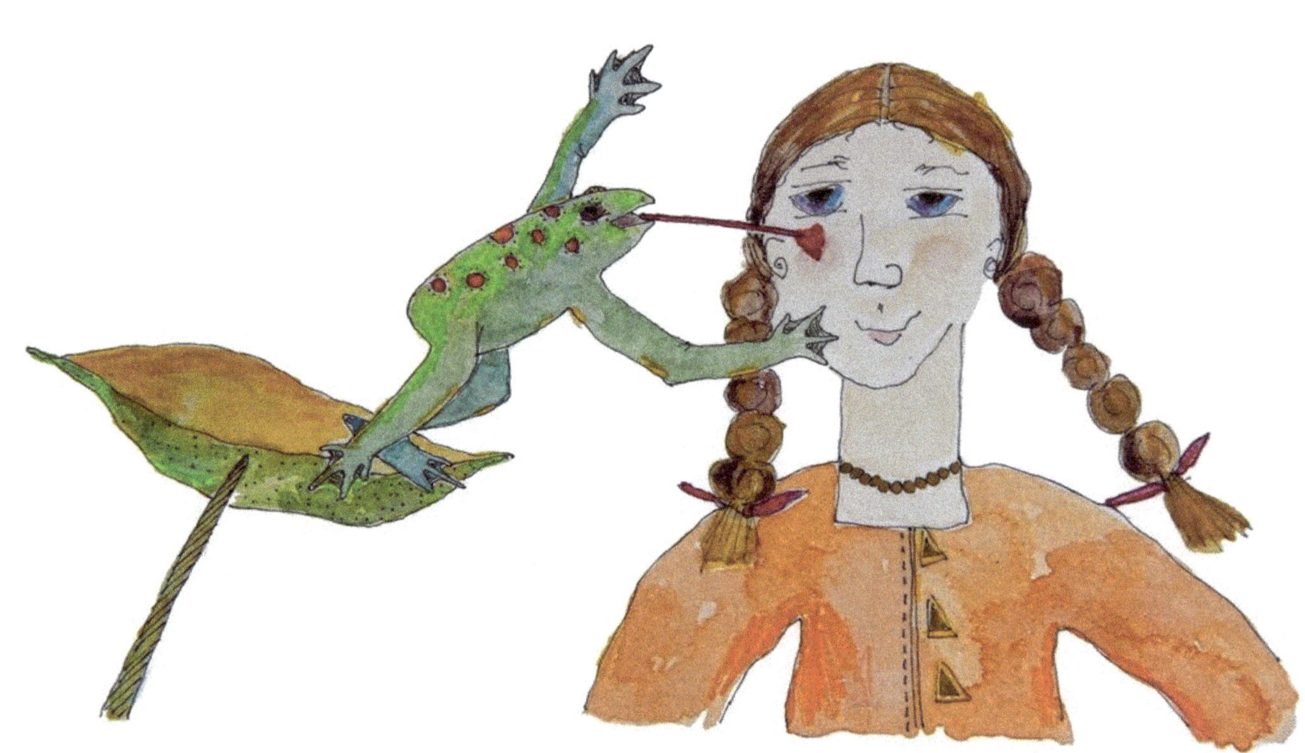

There are more tricks to learn about this, indeed.
Read on for more concepts to keep up to speed.

Strong feelings appeared with the mustard-less dogs.
Hurting back is not kind for humans or frogs.

It takes strength to chill out, give folks some slack.
Remember what goes out always boomerangs back.

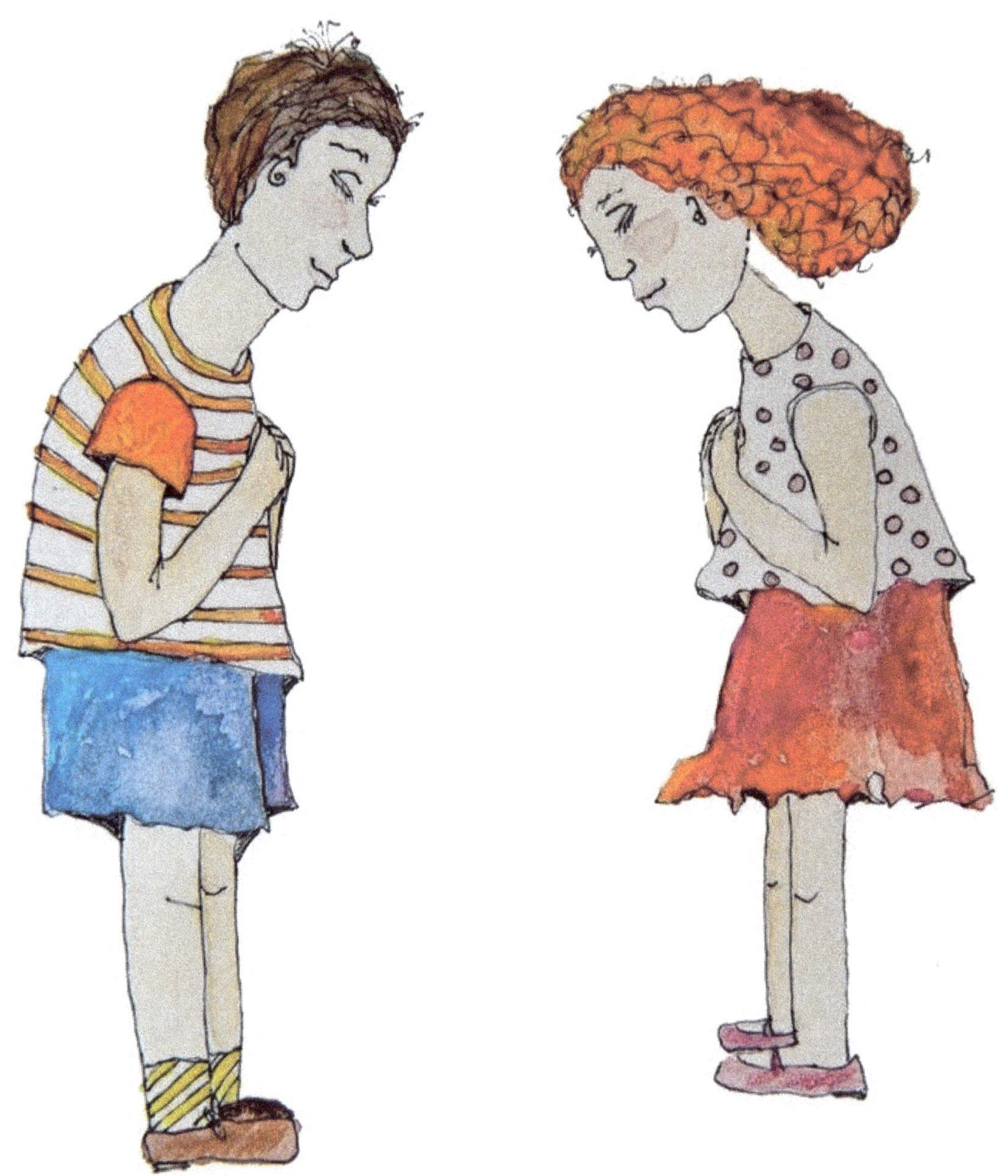

Differing opinions can be quite tough.

It's easy to be offended when vibes are rough.

If you're hurting it may help to look for some space,

'til you can share calmly, no scowl on your face.

We can dig in our heels and each stand our ground.

Yet, heartwarming ways can always be found.

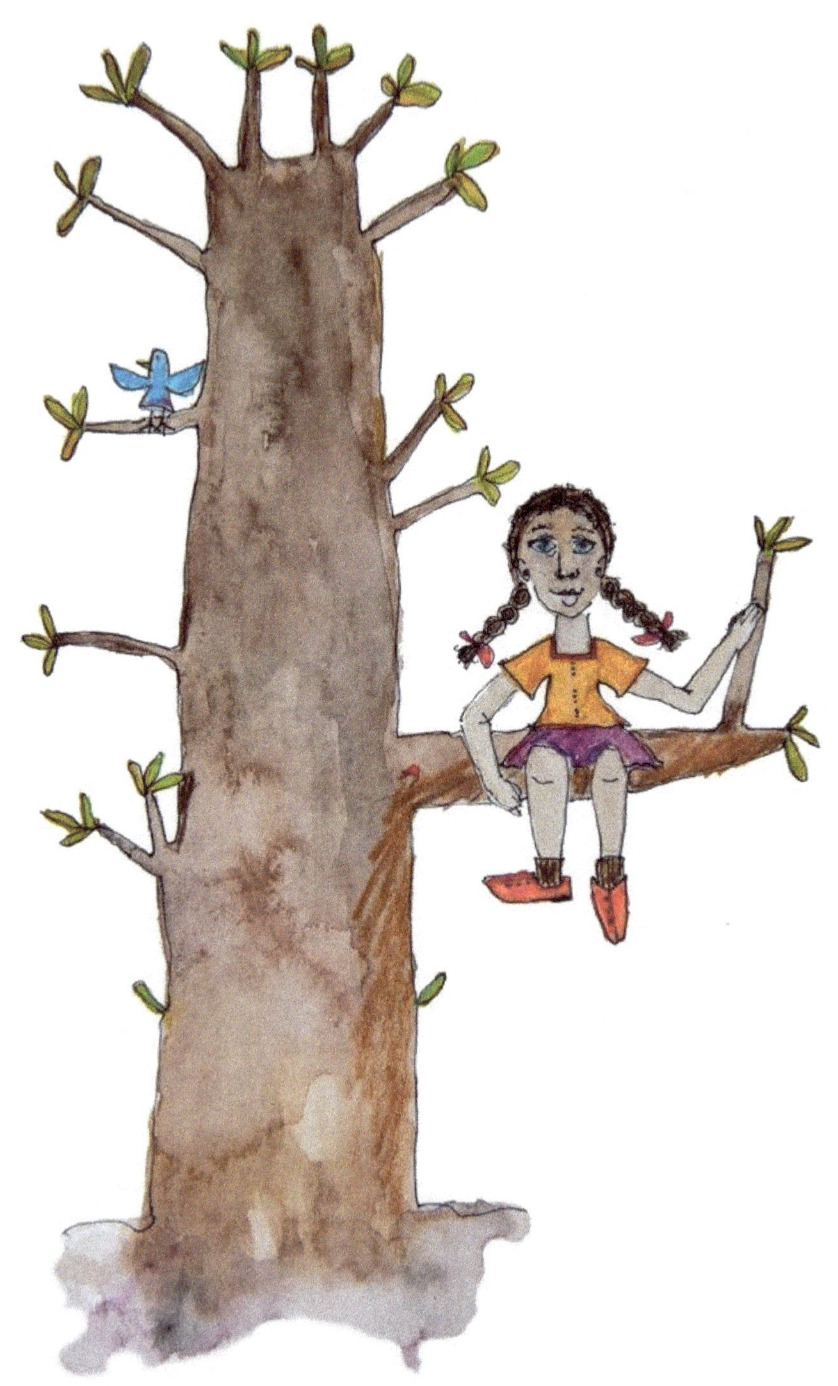

Trees are quite good with these types of endeavors.
Sit close to a tree 'til your anger surrenders.

Trees are well grounded and masters of breathing.
Imagine roots of your own to transmute your seething.

You could ask for help from a tree or a friend.
Wise ones know it's important for hearts to mend.

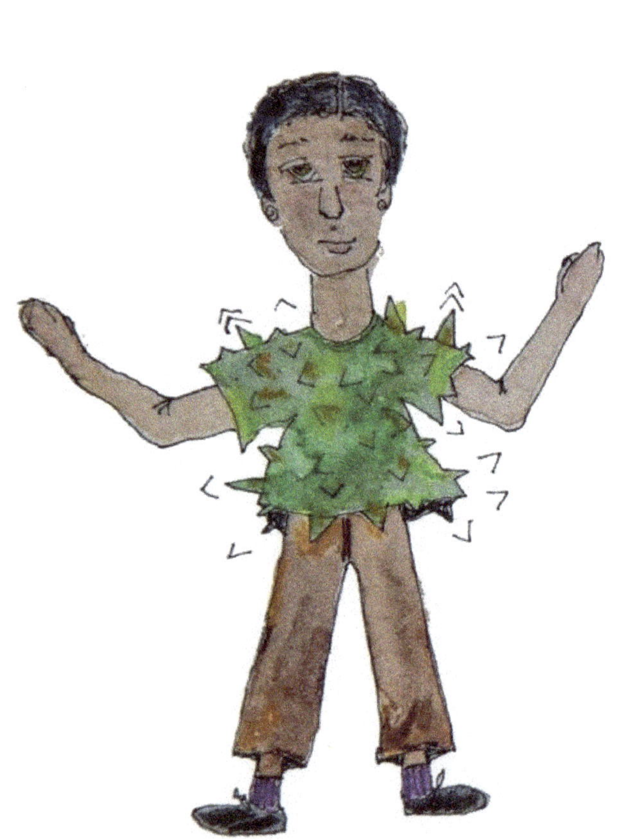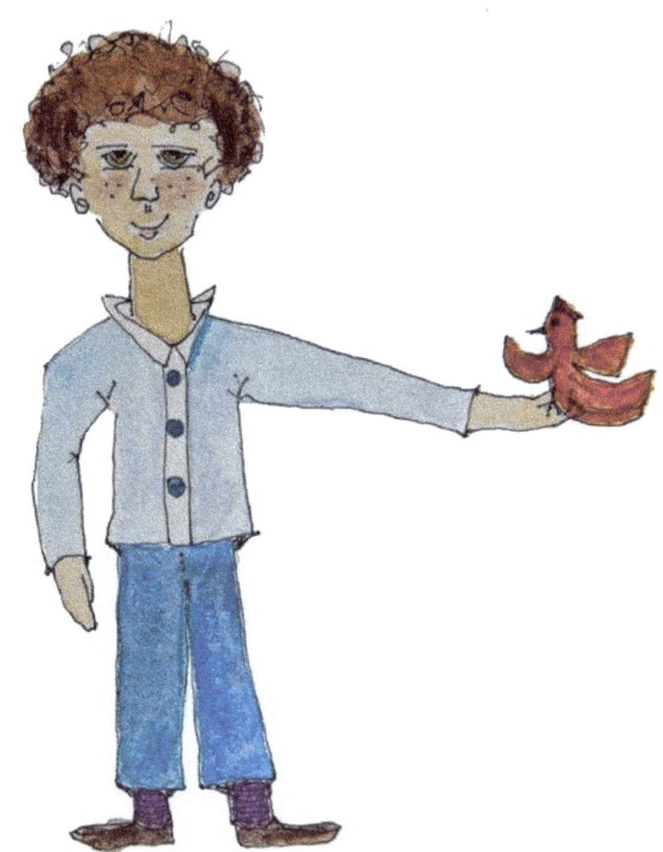

Reactions come fast, bringing thoughts of a duel.
Yes, we all can get back to keeping our cool.

Emotions are strong, and can happen quite quickly.
Compassion's not easy if you're feeling too prickly.

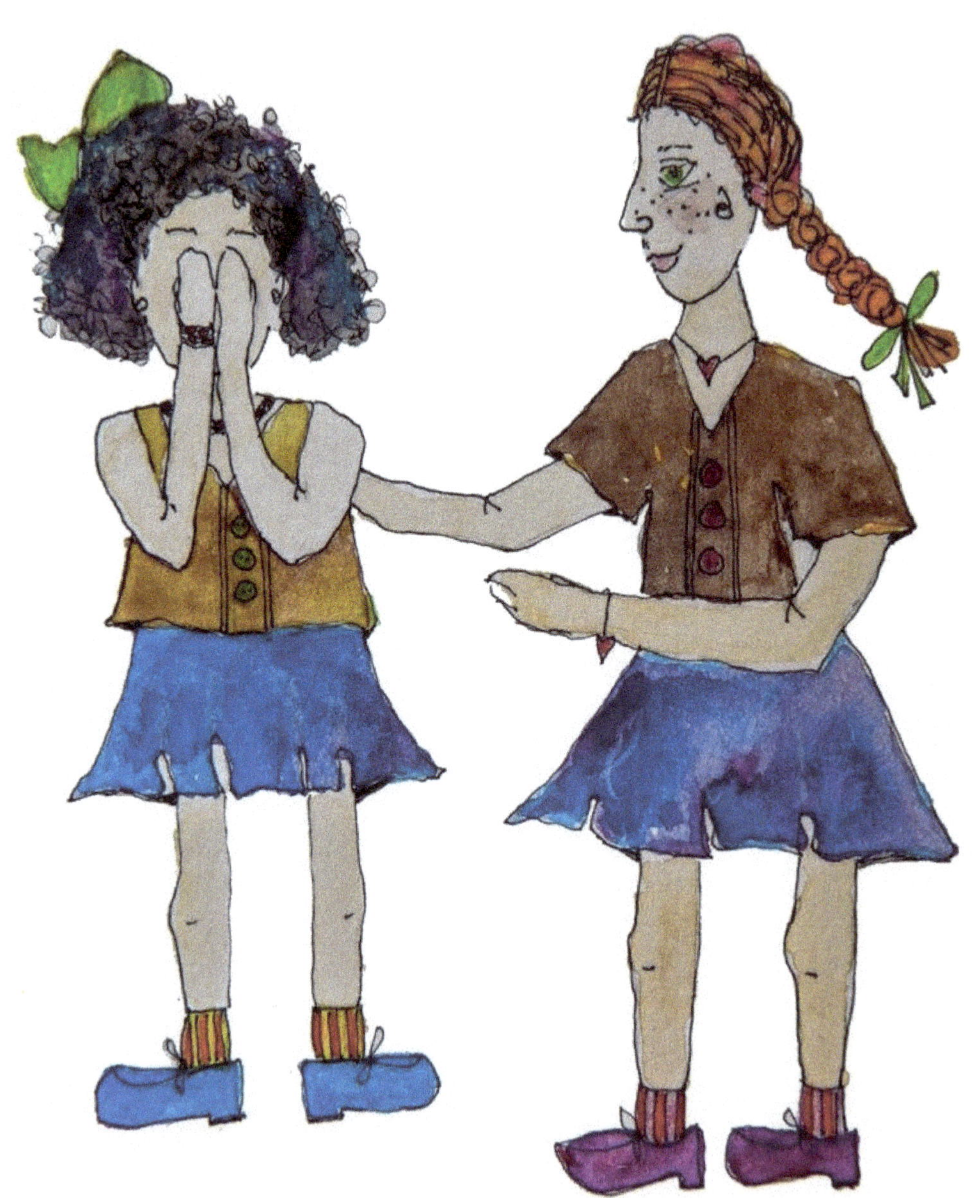

Expressing your feelings may help you unwind.
Sending 'arrows' to others is harmful, unkind.

Acting in anger usually has a big price.
Apologies can repair, are courteous, and quite nice.

Sad and mad feelings are normal when hurt.
Respect for each other helps to keep us alert.

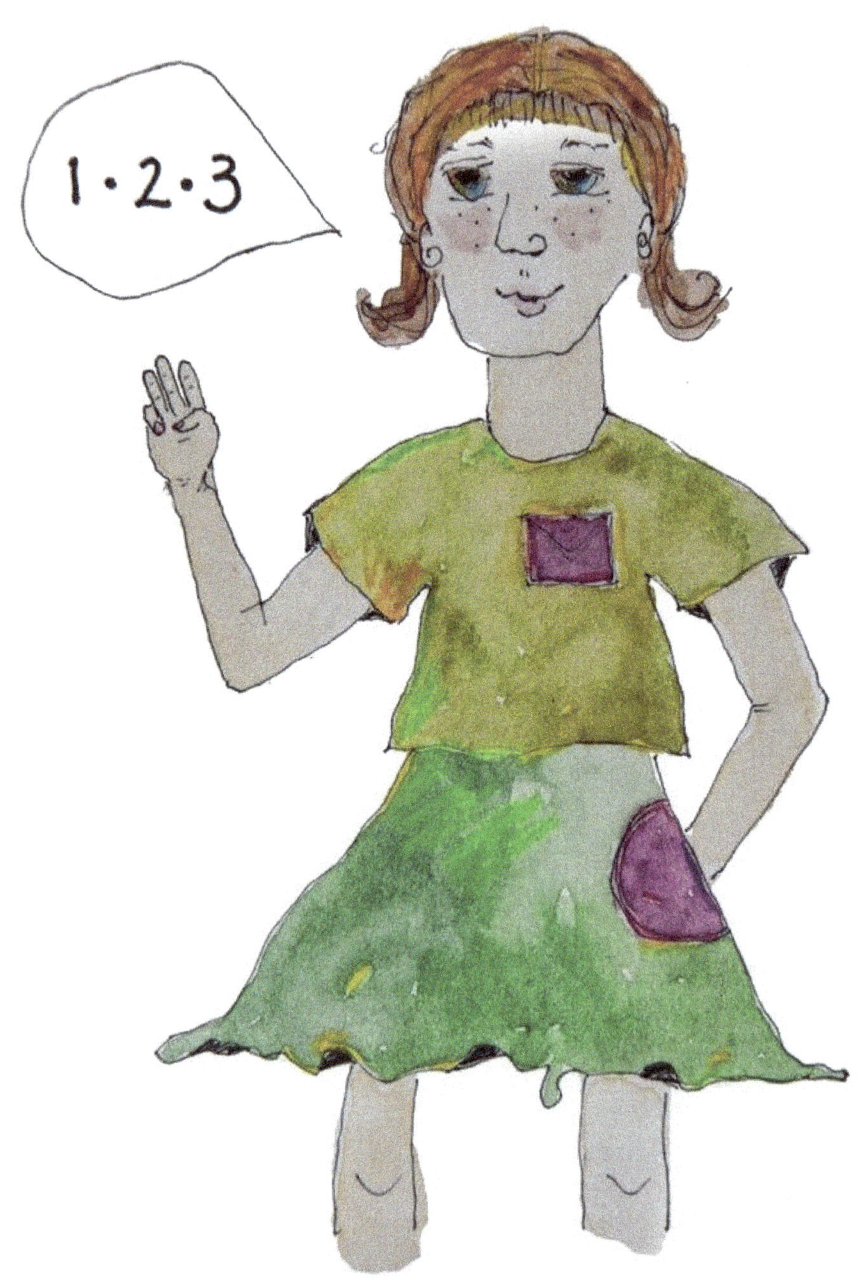
1·2·3

If you've let loose, quickly adjust, find your center.
Counting three breaths may help you remember.

You could shake like a dog when you're really upset,
Or you could sing, or dance, or play clarinet!

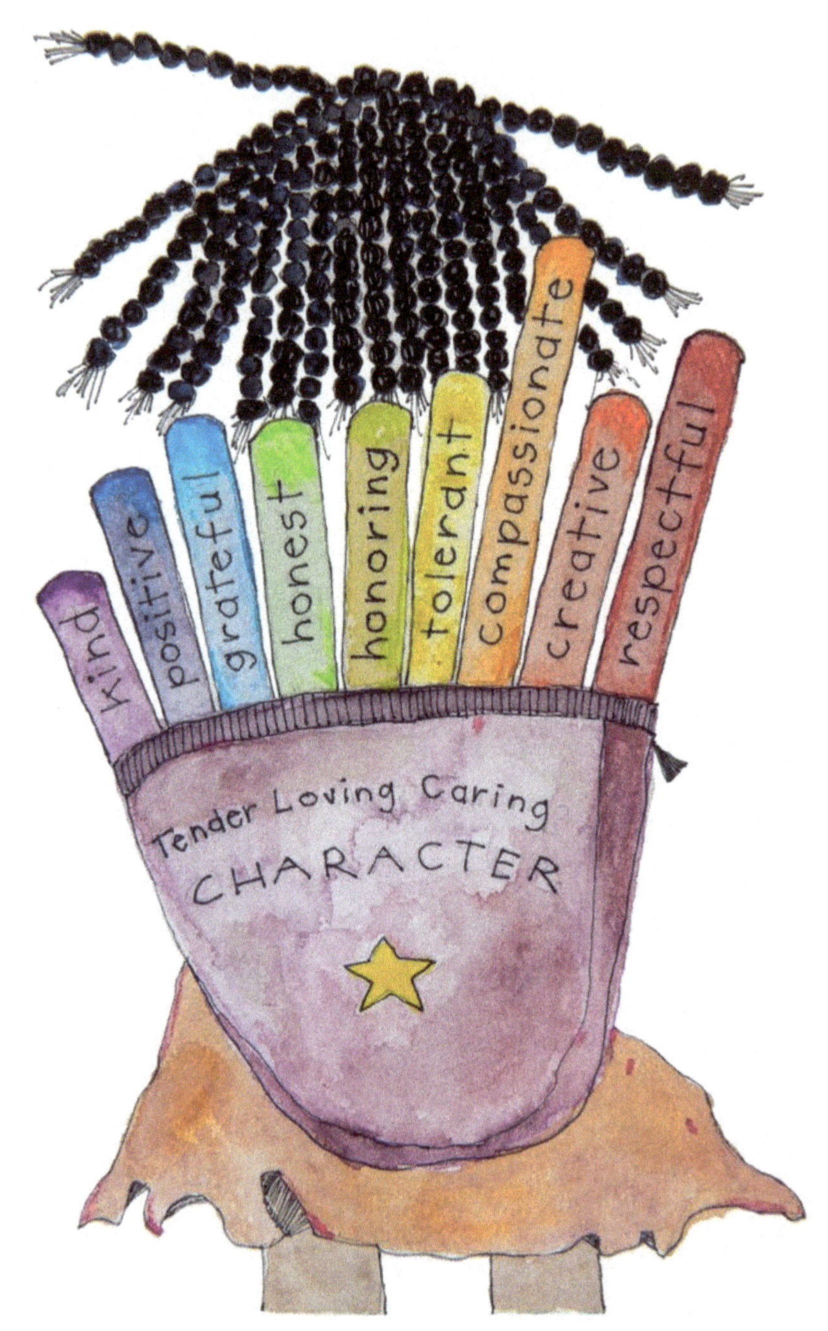

kind
positive
grateful
honest
honoring
tolerant
compassionate
creative
respectful
Tender Loving Caring
CHARACTER

Labels of good-bad, right-wrong add to the blame.
Thinking that way brings more violence and shame.

If you're speaking unkindly, wanting to hurt back.
You may need some TLC in your own knapsack.

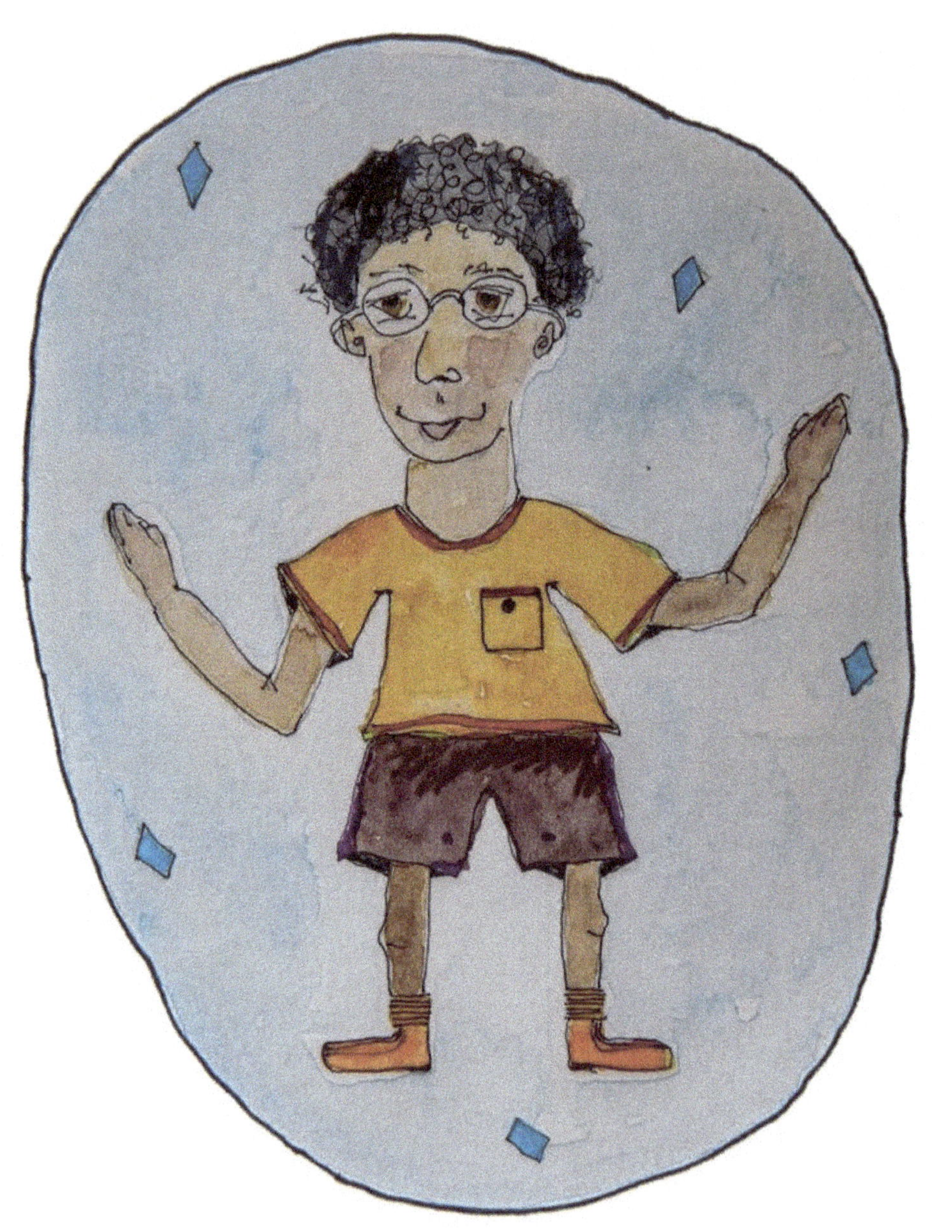

You aren't responsible for another's emotion.

It's their choice to get centered or make a commotion.

When you meet up with another who's ready to fight,

Wish them happiness or see them in a bubble of light.

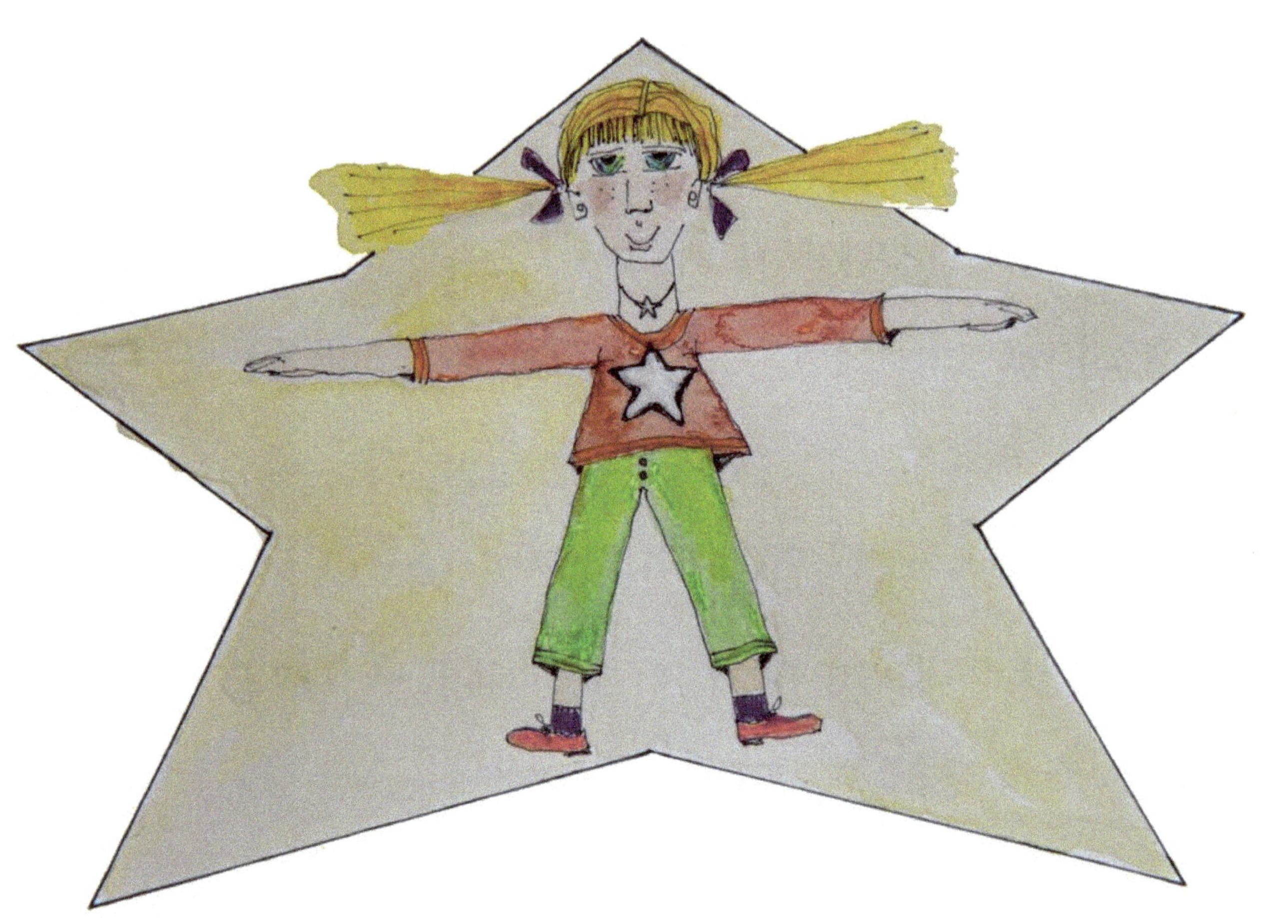

Others may seem to smoosh your experience.
Yet, only your response can pinch off your brilliance.

Those deep breaths of air help to soothe your mind.
Shining your starlight helps to keep you aligned.

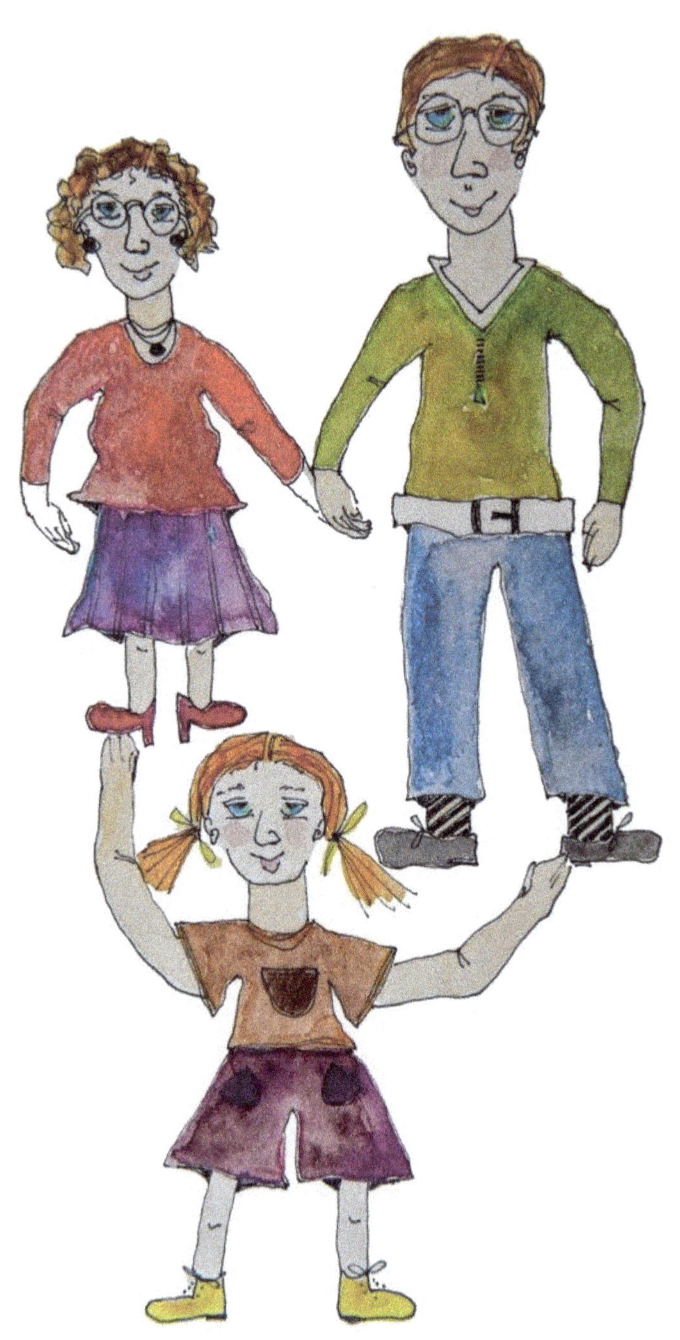

Life's disappointments bring us some sadness.
Choosing to calm helps to increase gladness.

Individuals and groups grow strong with this goal.
We light up the world when we find some control.

We all have a part in life's unique dances.
Owning our own emotion enhances.

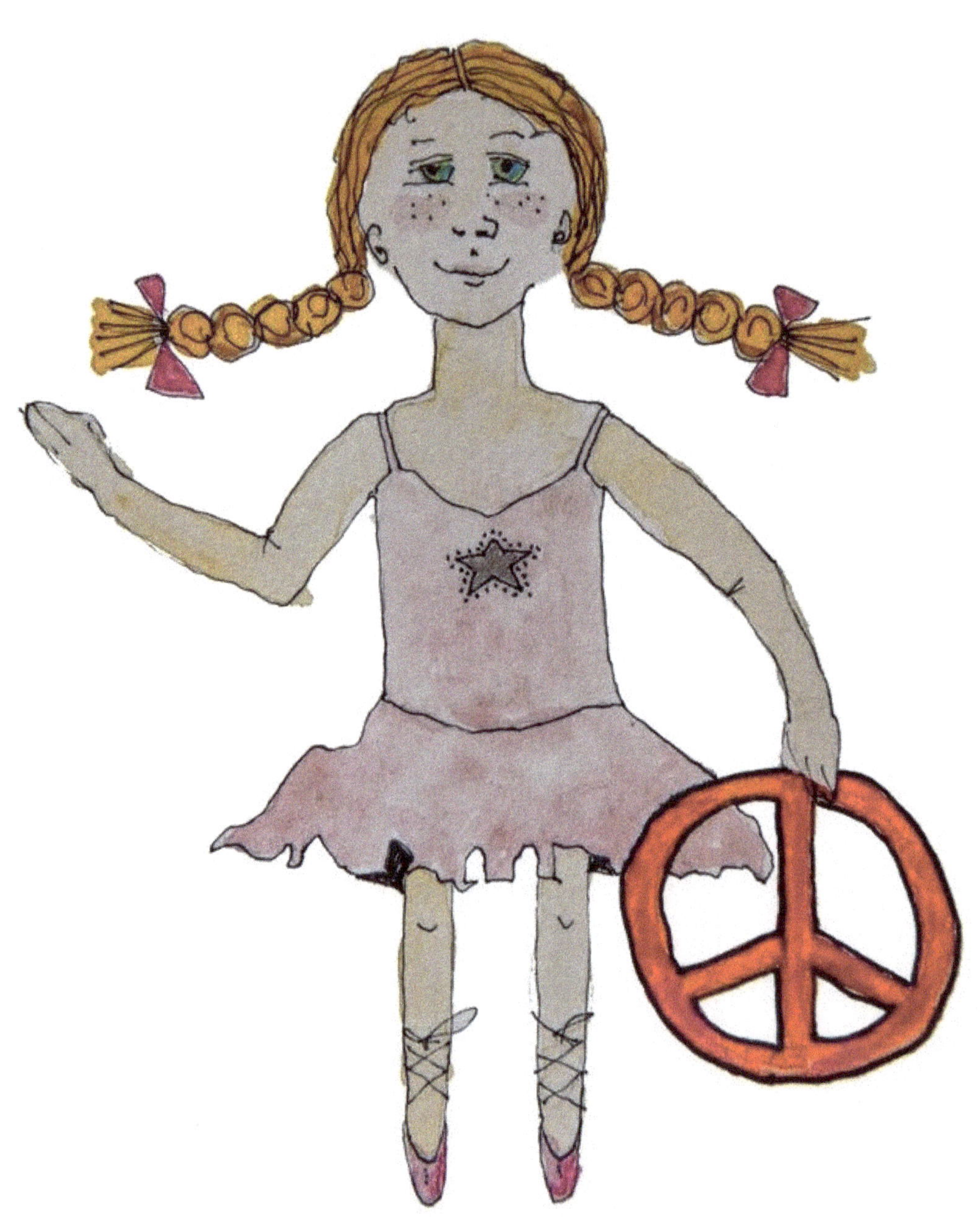

When worries or fears show up with full force,
Breathing with gratitude helps to change course.

There'll always be challenges in life, that's a given.
Would you be that someone to find peace within?

Show me a 'thumbs up' if you would, please,
Join other peacemakers across the seas!

Calming Breath Ideas
(10 minutes each day or whenever you need to calm or quiet your mind)

* Close your eyes. Breathe in slowly while silently counting: 1 – 2 – 3
  Breathe out slowly while silently counting: 1 – 2 – 3 – 4 – 5
  Feel and observe your breath going in and out of your lungs.

* Close your eyes. Breathe slowly at your own pace.
  Focus on the spaces in between each breath in and out.

* Close your eyes. Breathe slowly.
  As you breathe in imagine the air rising up inside your body
      from your feet up through the top of your head.
  As you breathe out imagine a waterfall of air going down
      the outside of your body from your head to your feet.

* Close your eyes.
  Slowly breathe in through your nose and out through your mouth.
  Feel your body expanding like a balloon. Release the air very quietly.
  With your mind's eye watch as the breaths fill you up and then go out.

* Close your eyes. Breathe in and out slowly.
  Imagine you are a tree breathing in and out, or see yourself
      filling up with sunlight, increasing it with each breath.
      Be a star shining bright.

Notable Quotes

The concepts in *Flustered Without Mustard* came from Brene' Brown's *Daring Greatly*, Esther Hicks' *Getting Into the Vortex Relationship Meditation*, Sandra Ingerman's *How to Heal Toxic Thoughts*, Harriet Lerner's *Dance of Anger*, and *Dance of Connection*, Marshall Rosenberg's *Non-Violent Communication*, and Marianne Williamson's *Return to Love*.

Brene' Brown

Daring Greatly: How the Courage to Be Vulnerable Transforms the Way We Live, Love, Parent, and Lead, Penguin Gotham Books (2012)

"What we know matters, but who we are matters more."

"Connection is why we're here; it is what gives purpose and meaning to our lives. The power that connection holds in our lives was confirmed when the main concern about connection emerged as the fear of disconnection; the fear that something we have done or failed to do, something about who we are or where we come from, has made us unlovable and unworthy of connection."

Esther Hicks, The Teachings of Abraham

Getting into the Vortex, Relationship Guided Meditation, Hay House, Inc. (2010)

"Sometimes it seems like others have the power to negatively affect your experience, but that is never true; only your response to them has the power to pinch you off from the naturally good-feeling person you are."

"Sometimes others believe that their happiness depends upon your response to them, but that is never true; and if you encourage them to believe that - and stand on your head to please them - you don't help them or you."

Sandra Ingerman

How to Heal Toxic Thoughts, Sterling Publishing Company, Inc. (2007)

"Think of a precious image. The energy behind your emotions goes out to all living beings."

Harriet Lerner

The Dance of Anger, Harper & Row, Publishers, Inc. (1985)

"Anger is a signal, and one worth listening to. Our anger may be a message that we are being hurt, that our rights are being violated, that our needs or wants are not being adequately met, or simply something is not right. Our anger may tell us that we are not addressing an important emotional issue in our lives, or that too much of our self - our beliefs, values, desires, or ambitions – is being compromised in a relationship."

'Anger is something we feel. It exists for a reason and always deserves our respect and attention. We all have a right to everything we feel - and certainly our anger is no exception.'

'There is, however, another side of the coin: If feeling angry signals a problem, venting anger does not solve it. Those of us who are locked into ineffective expressions of anger suffer as deeply as those of us who dare not get angry at all.'

The Dance of Connection, HarperCollins Publishers (2001)

'...establish some ground rules for fighting rather than assuming that feeling enraged ('I can't help myself') gives you license to say or do anything. If you can't maintain control of your own voice, you need professional help.' [This book includes Dr. Gottman's relationship disasters and repair attempts too.]

Marshall Rosenberg

Non-Violent Communication: A Language of Life, PuddleDancer Press (2015)

'I see all anger as a result of life-alienating, violence-provoking thinking. At the core of all anger is a need that is not being fulfilled. Thus anger can be valuable if we use it as an alarm clock to wake us up - to realize we have a need that isn't being met and that we are thinking in a way that makes it unlikely to be met.

'...to fully express anger requires full consciousness of our need. In addition, energy is required to get the need met. Anger, however, co-opts our energy by directing it toward punishing people rather than meeting our needs. Instead of engaging in 'righteous indignation,' I recommend connecting empathically with our own needs or those of others. This may take extensive practice, whereby over and over again, we consciously replace the phrase 'I am angry because they .....' with 'I am angry because I am needing .....''

'The four steps to expressing anger are (1) stop and breathe, (2) identify our judgmental thoughts, (3) connect with our needs, and (4) express our feelings and unmet needs. Sometimes, in between steps 3 and 4, we may choose to empathize with the other person so that he or she will be better able to hear us when we express ourselves in step 4.

Marianne Williamson

A Return to Love, Harper One (1992)

'Ego says, 'Once everything falls into place, I'll feel peace.' Spirit says, 'Find your peace, and then everything will fall into place.''

Testimonials

Administrators & Teachers
Jackie Burt, Founder of Orsch, a Fabulous School and Educational Philosophy

Flustered Without Mustard: Finding Calm When Angry or Frustrated is a beautiful reminder to source inner peace, which is often easier said than done. It offers a variety of options and go-to solutions that heal and calm in times of need. This is the type of book that can be read over and over again, and continue to serve with its messages of true mindfulness and loving energy. A book for all ages and all humans.

Susan Conroy, Ph.D. Administration, Principal & Music Teacher

Flustered Without Mustard sets a stage for discussion with 'kids' of any age - 1 to 100. While the clever topic of mustard on a hot dog is quite simple, discussion on the range of reactions is not simple. Finding ways to resolve conflicts causing anger or frustration are as important as reading and math, for if emotions are not successfully mastered, success in academics will be hampered and relationships will struggle. Thank you for your creative ways, Barbara. You are a treasure to the world of ideas and solutions.

Sonia Fuderer, MA Education, Literacy Interventionist, KY

In a time when mindfulness is making its way into classrooms around the world, *Flustered Without Mustard: Finding Calm When Angry or Frustrated* shows children the tools they need to handle varying emotional situations in a kid-friendly, beautifully illustrated book that will foster beneficial conversations at home and in the classroom.

Nan Gaylen, Ph.D. Educational Administration & Policy, IL

Flustered Without Mustard: Finding Calm When Angry or Frustrated could be used as a wonderful teaching tool in facilitating a discussion with young students regarding how to personally respond to situations we find stressful in our world today. There are so many possibilities for use in a classroom, only some of which may be writing, telling, painting, singing, or acting out our own ways of showing kindness, calmness, and inner strength.

Minda Morren López, Ph.D. Culture, Language, & Literacy, Associate Professor of Literacy, Texas State University, TX

Flustered Without Mustard: Finding Calm When Angry or Frustrated is a wonderful book with beautiful illustrations that can be used by parents and educators alike to build empathy and support socio-emotional learning. The first part of the book takes an extremely relatable event from various perspectives and gives readers a way to respond to disappointment that is healthy and intentional. The second part of the book expands outward to broader themes and experiences that all human beings can relate to while providing ways to center ourselves, take responsibility for our own behaviors, and respond positively to challenging situations. The practical suggestions for calming breaths could be used by all ages in a variety of contexts.

As a mother, teacher, and teacher educator, I will use this book as part of guiding children through understanding and naming emotions, and responding in healthy ways to the messiness of life as we go through it. Thank you, Barbara and Mary Ann, for a wonderful book that is a welcome addition to children's texts that support mindfulness and socio-emotional regulation and health. We need more books like this that support such important work.

Kelly Piccaro, MA Education, Kindergarten Teacher, CO

Flustered Without Mustard: Finding Calm When Angry or Frustrated is a wonderful book that speaks to any age. We all have those days and those moments when something unexpected happens, something not up to our standard or our liking. It is how we choose to respond and how we treat those people around us that truly show our character. This book helps us see how people identify with their problem and choose to react.

Personally and professionally, as a Kindergarten teacher, I love the specific emotions and colorful words used in the story. The language helps children identify and grapple with their own feelings and develop new skills for moving forward as they negotiate their own world.

Becky Thornburg, MA Administration, Teacher & Principal, CO

How many times have you been disappointed when you were expecting some mustard, and there was none? Life is a series of challenges and reactions. Author, Barbara, and illustrator, Mary Ann, have shared a lively story of how various hot dog shoppers reacted to bad news.

Flustered Without Mustard offers an abundance of ideas, which suggests that being loving and positive may indeed outnumber and be of greater benefit to all concerned than the alternatives. Each choice is worthy of discussion between parent and child or teacher and students. Don't stop with discussion. Encourage activities: art, posters, dramatics, and writing.

Whether it's mustard or custard that is missing today.
You can be mad, sad, or refuse to play.
Or maybe, if you remember this tale,
Other actions more calming and kind will prevail.

Artists
Dale Payson, Artist & Children's Book Illustrator, NY

I have to say I LOVE the illustrations in *Flustered Without Mustard: Finding Calm When Angry or Frustrated*. They are so honest, and delightfully childlike. I truly believe the art is wonderful and people of any age will connect favorably to it!

Authors
Imelda Almqvist, International Teacher of Sacred Art and Northern European Shamanism; Author of *Natural Born Shamans: A Spiritual Toolkit For Life* and *Sacred Art: A Hollow Bone for Spirit*, and *Medicine of the Imagination: Dwelling in Possibility*, UK

Barbara Haas is one of the most gifted and inspiring educators I know. She is positively electric! The child in her sings and dances with all children, and ex-children, who cross her path. She makes learning fun and her book *Flustered Without Mustard: Finding Calm When Angry or Frustrated* offers positive ways of dealing with tricky situations, an art all human children need to master!

In my mother tongue, Dutch, Haas means 'hare' and I can't help seeing delightful glimpses of a hare hopping all over the globe delivering this book to the children and families who need it! I urge you to read this book and dance with Barbara 'Rhubarb' Haas!

Kathleen T. Pelley, Children's Author, *The Giant King*, and *Inventor McGregor*, and *Magnus Maximus, A Marvelous Measurer*, and others, CO

Flustered Without Mustard: Finding Calm When Angry or Frustrated is a fun fable for kids and adults that shares some great insights on how to cope with anger and frustration by tapping into our inner light and strength. This would make a great introduction to meditation and mindfulness for kids (and maybe some adults too). It is certainly a welcome tonic for our world today as we strive to teach children kindness, and how to get along with each other despite our differences.

Counselors
Sophie Bloch-Miller, Licensed Clinical Social Worker, OR

Flustered Without Mustard: Finding Calm When Angry or Frustrated captures the range of emotional and behavioral responses that individuals, young and old, have when met with disappointment and frustration. This book does a lovely job of introducing and modeling coping skills for managing emotions, while considering the harmful impact to self and others when we simply react, rather than self soothe and regulate our emotional response. Barbara provides examples of somatic coping skills such as deep breathing, as well as social and cognitive coping skills to help redirect one's focus from the distressing event to more positive points of focus.

This book is a great resource for the classroom, the therapy office, or the home. It offers tools to help children normalize their own emotional experiences, and a range of choices to build healthy character and emotional well being.

Sara Lamar, MA, Licensed School Counselor, CO

As a middle school counselor, I am always looking for new and creative ways to advocate for and support my students. The moment I finished reading *Flustered Without Mustard: Finding Calm When Angry or Frustrated* I knew that I had found a gem that will be in my toolbox for many years to come! We all have those days where unexpected challenges could derail our hopes and our goals, and we all react to stress in different ways.

I love how Barbara has provided multiple coping strategies for calming down and Mary Ann's wonderful illustrations allow all types of learners to connect with the teachings embedded within the book. It shows that we can all make mistakes and overcome them with positivity, growth, and resilience. This is a wonderful book for all ages, and I will definitely be incorporating it into my school counseling curriculum as well as reading it with my family!

Former 5th Grade Student
Whitney Schmidt Amaral, Television & Film
Production Designer & Graphic Designer

Mrs. Haas influenced me greatly as an elementary school student, and had a profound impact on the creative person I am today. It's inspiring to see her put her talent and passion for teaching into a book that helps students of all levels learn how to cope with the challenges life brings. The delightful and insightful *Flustered Without Mustard* will leave a positive impact on all who read it.

Parents, students, teachers, and counselors, we'd love to hear from you!
We would like to share your testimonials on our Rhubarb Wisdom Books' website.
Please send your comments and anecdotes to: RhubarbWisdomBooks@gmail.com
Thank you for recommending this book to your friends, family, schools, and libraries!

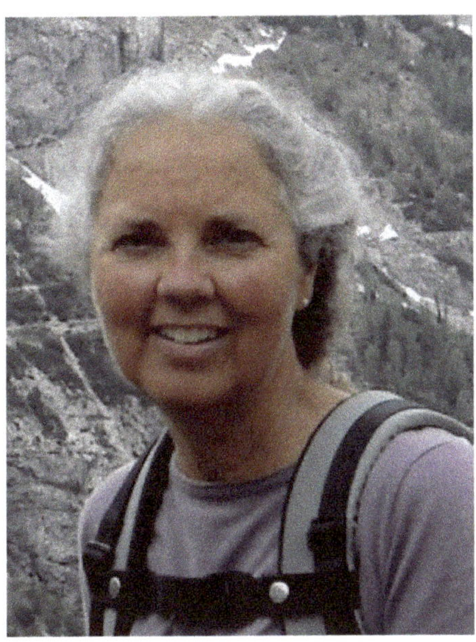 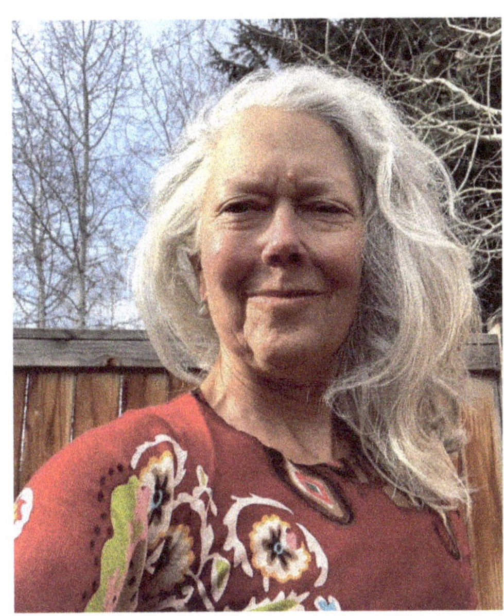

About the Author:

Barbara 'Rhubarb' Haas lives in Colorado's Rocky Mountains with her husband, Chris, and their furry feline, Frank. She has been in the education field from the Madeline Hunter to the Kagan & Kagan eras, has taught many ages and many subjects, spending most of her career with 5th graders. She honed her writing skills for her Masters in Education, and courses beyond that, as well as grant writing for her Artists-in-Residence programs. She has had several articles and poems published, and is delighted to share this latest adventure in word wranglin'.

About the Illustrator:

Mary Ann Kruse, June Hog Designs, is recognized for her vibrant watercolor depictions of wildlife created with illustrative authenticity and a hint of artistic license for creative engagement. Fishes, birds, and bees are her usual subjects with their exceptional texture and hues, scales, feathers and fur. Honoring wildlife in their essential roles and paying tribute to their exquisite beauty, she now adds humans to her whimsical artwork. She lives with two felines, Ursa and Zubenelgenubi (aka Zube) in Oregon's high desert where the scent of sage meets gnarled juniper.